HEALING HERBAL TEA BIBLE:

Master the Art of Preparing Nourishing Infusions to Promote Wellness and Vitality

BY

SARAH PARTISON

TABLE OF CONTENTS

INTRODUCTION

Welcome to the enchanting world of herbal teas, where the delicate dance of leaves and petals transforms into a soothing elixir that not only tantalizes the taste buds but also nurtures the body and soul. In the midst of our fast-paced lives, the Healing Herbal Tea Bible beckons you to rediscover the age-old tradition of herbal tea crafting, a practice that transcends time and culture.

Within the pages of this comprehensive guide, you will embark on a journey through the verdant landscapes of nature's pharmacy, exploring the vast array of herbs and botanicals that have been revered for their healing properties for centuries. The Healing Herbal Tea Bible is not just a compendium of recipes; it is a celebration of the ancient wisdom that has been passed down through generations, offering you a holistic approach to well-being.

As you delve into the pages of this botanical treasure trove, you will discover the art and science behind blending herbs to create teas that address a myriad of health concerns. From soothing chamomile to invigorating peppermint, each herb tells a story of healing, providing a natural remedy for ailments that have plagued humanity for generations. Whether you seek relaxation, immunity support, or a rejuvenating energy boost, the Healing Herbal Tea Bible is your guide to unlocking the therapeutic potential of plants.

But this book is more than just a collection of recipes—it's a guide to understanding the alchemy of herbal infusions. Learn about the unique properties of herbs, their traditional uses, and how to harness their full potential through proper preparation. Immerse yourself in the world of tisanes, decoctions, and infusions, and discover the nuances of flavor, aroma, and health benefits that each cup holds.

With expert advice on sourcing, drying, and storing herbs, as well as detailed instructions for creating your own personalized blends, the Healing Herbal Tea Bible empowers you to become a master tea alchemist in your own kitchen. Whether you are a seasoned herbalist or a curious beginner, this book provides a roadmap to cultivating a deeper connection with nature and embracing the therapeutic power of plants.

So, join us on this aromatic voyage, where the Healing Herbal Tea Bible becomes your trusted companion on the path to well-being. Let the steam rise from your cup, carrying with it the essence of centuries-old wisdom and the promise of a healthier, more balanced life. Cheers to the ancient art of herbal tea, where healing meets harmony in every sip.

CHAPTER 1: GETTING STARTED WITH HERBAL TEAS

Understanding Different Types of Herbs

Herbal teas have been cherished for centuries, celebrated not only for their diverse flavors but also for their potential health benefits. Whether you're a tea enthusiast or a newcomer to the world of herbal infusions, understanding the different types of herbs used in herbal teas is a fascinating journey that can enhance your overall well-being.

1. Chamomile: The Calming Elixir

Chamomile is renowned for its calming properties. Often consumed before bedtime, chamomile tea helps to relax the mind and body, promoting a restful sleep. This gentle herb also aids in digestion, making it an excellent choice after a meal.

2. Peppermint: Refreshingly Invigorating

Peppermint tea is a popular choice for its refreshing and invigorating qualities. Known for its ability to soothe the digestive system, alleviate headaches, and provide a burst of energy, peppermint tea is a versatile herb that can be enjoyed both hot and cold.

3. Lavender: A Fragrant Relaxation

Lavender isn't just for aromatherapy; it can also be a delightful addition to your tea collection. Lavender tea is celebrated for its calming effects, helping to alleviate stress and anxiety. Its fragrant aroma adds a touch of tranquility to your tea-drinking experience.

4. Ginger: Warming and Soothing

Ginger tea is a warming infusion that is both flavorful and beneficial. Known for its anti-inflammatory properties, ginger tea can help soothe an upset stomach, alleviate nausea, and provide comfort during colder seasons. Its spicy kick adds a zesty note to your cup.

5. Hibiscus: Vibrant and Tart

Hibiscus tea, made from the dried petals of the hibiscus flower, boasts a vibrant crimson hue and a tart flavor profile. Rich in antioxidants, hibiscus tea is known for promoting heart health and may help lower blood pressure. Enjoy it hot or cold for a refreshing experience.

6. Rooibos: South African Delight

Rooibos, or red bush tea, is a caffeine-free herbal tea native to South Africa. Its earthy, slightly sweet taste makes it a popular choice for those seeking a caffeine-free alternative. Rooibos is also rich in antioxidants, contributing to its potential health benefits.

7. Dandelion: Detoxifying Brew

Dandelion tea is not only a great way to put those backyard weeds to use but also a powerful detoxifying brew. Believed to support liver health, dandelion tea has a slightly bitter taste that can be balanced with a touch of honey or lemon.

8. Nettle: Nutrient-Rich Infusion

Nettle tea, made from the leaves of the stinging nettle plant, is a nutrient-rich herbal infusion. It is believed to have anti-inflammatory properties and may provide relief for seasonal allergies. Nettle tea has a mild, earthy flavor and can be enjoyed on its own or blended with other herbs.

Tips for Brewing Herbal Teas:

Water Temperature: Use freshly boiled water, but be mindful of the temperature. Delicate herbs like chamomile and mint benefit from slightly cooler water, around 190°F (88°C), while heartier herbs like ginger can withstand boiling water.

Steeping Time: Allow the herbs to steep for 5-10 minutes, depending on the type of herb and your desired strength of flavor. Longer steeping times may intensify the taste.

Experiment with Blends: Don't hesitate to create your own herbal tea blends. Mixing different herbs can result in unique and personalized flavor profiles.

Sweeteners and Enhancements: Feel free to add honey, lemon, or other natural sweeteners to enhance the flavor of your herbal tea. Experiment until you find the perfect combination for your taste buds.

Embark on your herbal tea journey by exploring the vast array of herbs available. Whether you're seeking relaxation, a burst of energy, or specific health benefits, the world of herbal teas offers a diverse and delightful array of options.

Selecting High-Quality Ingredients

Herbal teas have been cherished for centuries for their delightful flavors and potential health benefits. Whether you're a seasoned tea enthusiast or a newcomer to the world of herbal infusions, the key to a satisfying cup lies in selecting high-quality ingredients. In this guide, we'll explore the essentials of getting started with herbal teas, emphasizing the importance of choosing premium herbs for a truly exceptional tea experience.

Understanding Herbal Teas:

Herbal teas, also known as tisanes, are caffeine-free infusions made from a variety of dried flowers, leaves, seeds, and roots. Unlike true teas, which are derived from the Camellia sinensis plant, herbal teas provide a diverse range of flavors, aromas, and potential health benefits. Before embarking on your herbal tea journey, it's crucial to understand the properties and uses of different herbs.

Selecting High-Quality Herbs:
The quality of your herbal tea starts with the ingredients you choose. When selecting herbs, consider the following factors:

a. Organic and Sustainably Sourced: Opt for organic herbs to minimize exposure to pesticides and ensure a more natural flavor profile. Additionally, choosing sustainably sourced herbs supports ethical and environmentally friendly practices.

b. Freshness: Freshness is key to the potency of herbal teas. Look for herbs that are vibrant in color, aromatic, and free from signs of staleness or mold.

c. Whole Leaf vs. Cut and Sifted: Whole leaf herbs often maintain their essential oils and flavors better than cut and sifted varieties. However, both options can yield excellent teas depending on personal preferences.

d. Appearance and Aroma: Inspect the appearance and aroma of the herbs. High-quality herbs should have a robust fragrance and vibrant colors. Avoid herbs that appear dull or lack aroma.

Popular Herbal Tea Ingredients:

Explore a variety of herbs to create unique and personalized herbal tea blends. Some popular choices include:

a. Peppermint: Refreshing and known for its digestive properties.

b. Chamomile: Calming and perfect for relaxation before bedtime.

c. Lavender: Delicate and floral, often used for relaxation and stress relief.

d. Ginger: Warming and spicy, with potential digestive benefits.

e. Hibiscus: Tart and vibrant, rich in antioxidants.

Blending Your Own Herbal Teas:

Once you've gathered a selection of high-quality herbs, experiment with creating your own blends. Combine complementary flavors and experiment with different ratios to find the perfect balance. Consider adding dried fruits, spices, or other herbs to enhance the complexity of your blends.

Brewing Tips:

Brewing herbal teas is a simple yet nuanced process. Here are some general tips to ensure a flavorful cup:

a. Water Temperature: Use boiling water for most herbal teas, but avoid using water that's too hot for delicate herbs like chamomile or hibiscus.

b. Steeping Time: Herbal teas generally require a longer steeping time than traditional teas. Allow your herbs to steep for 5-7 minutes or longer, depending on personal preference.

c. Experiment: Feel free to experiment with steeping times, water temperatures, and herb combinations to discover your preferred flavor profile.

Getting started with herbal teas is a delightful journey into the world of natural flavors and potential health benefits. By selecting high-quality ingredients, understanding the properties of different herbs, and experimenting with blends, you can create a customized tea experience that suits your taste preferences. Embrace the art of herbal tea crafting and savor the rich tapestry of flavors that nature has to offer.

Essential Tools and Equipment for Herbal Tea Preparation

The world of herbal teas is not only a delightful experience for your taste buds but also a step towards embracing the therapeutic benefits of various herbs and botanicals. To ensure a seamless and enjoyable herbal tea preparation process, it's essential to have the right tools and equipment at your disposal. In this guide, we'll explore the key items you need to get started with brewing your own herbal teas.

Tea Infusers:

One of the fundamental tools for preparing herbal teas is a reliable tea infuser. These come in various forms, such as ball infusers, basket infusers, and disposable tea bags. Choose an infuser that suits your preference and makes it easy to steep your favorite herbs without the mess.

Teapots or Tea Kettles:

A good quality teapot or tea kettle is essential for brewing herbal teas. Opt for materials like glass, ceramic, or stainless steel to avoid any interference with the flavors of your herbs. Electric kettles with temperature control are particularly handy for achieving the perfect steeping temperature for different herbs.

Mortar and Pestle:

For those who enjoy using whole herbs and spices in their tea blends, a mortar and pestle are invaluable tools. Grinding herbs just before brewing releases their essential oils, intensifying the flavors and aromas in your tea.

Herb Scissors:

Herb scissors are designed with multiple blades to efficiently chop herbs for tea blends. They make the process quicker and more precise compared to using a regular knife, ensuring an even distribution of flavors in your herbal infusions.

Measuring Tools:

Accurate measurements are crucial for achieving the perfect balance of flavors in your herbal teas. Invest in measuring spoons or a kitchen scale to portion your herbs correctly and create consistently delicious blends.

Storage Containers:

Proper storage is essential to preserve the freshness and potency of your herbs. Use airtight containers made of glass or metal to shield your herbs from light, air, and moisture. Label each container with the herb's name and expiration date to stay organized.

Water Filtration System:

The quality of water you use significantly impacts the taste of your herbal tea. Consider using filtered or spring water to enhance the purity of your brew. A water filtration system can remove impurities and provide a clean canvas for your herbal infusions.

Thermometer:

Maintaining the right steeping temperature is crucial for extracting the full flavor and benefits of herbs. A kitchen thermometer will help you monitor water temperature, ensuring that you steep delicate herbs at lower temperatures and hardier ones at higher temperatures.

Timer:

Steeping times vary for different herbs, and oversteeping can lead to bitter flavors. Use a timer to keep track of the brewing time and achieve a perfect balance in your herbal teas.

Equipping yourself with the essential tools for herbal tea preparation sets the foundation for a delightful and rewarding experience. As you explore the diverse world of herbs and their unique flavors, these tools will become your trusted companions, enabling you to craft personalized blends that cater to your taste and well-being. So, gather your equipment, select your favorite herbs, and embark on a journey of aromatic and flavorful herbal tea exploration.

CHAPTER 2: THE ART OF BLENDING

Basic Principles of Herbal Tea Blending

The world of herbal tea is a delightful journey of flavors, aromas, and therapeutic benefits. One of the key elements that contribute to the richness of herbal teas is the art of blending. Herbal tea blending is a nuanced practice that involves combining various herbs, flowers, fruits, and spices to create a harmonious and well-balanced infusion. Understanding the basic principles of herbal tea blending allows enthusiasts to craft unique blends that cater to personal preferences and health goals.

Selecting Base Herbs:

The foundation of any herbal tea blend is the base herb or herbs. These are the primary ingredients that provide the overall character and properties of the tea. Common base herbs include chamomile, peppermint, lemongrass, and hibiscus. Choose base herbs based on the desired flavor profile and potential health benefits.

Balancing Flavors:

Achieving a well-balanced flavor is a fundamental aspect of herbal tea blending. Consider the taste profile of each herb—some may be sweet, others earthy, while some are more pungent or spicy. By combining herbs with complementary flavors, you can create a blend that is neither too overpowering nor too subtle. Experiment with different ratios to find the perfect balance.

Adding Aromatic Herbs:

Aromatic herbs such as lavender, rose petals, and mint can elevate the sensory experience of herbal teas. These herbs contribute fragrant notes that enhance the overall aroma of the blend. A well-thought-out combination of aromatic herbs can turn a simple cup of tea into a sensory delight.

Incorporating Fruits and Citrus:

Dried fruits like berries, citrus peels, or apple pieces can add a touch of sweetness and tanginess to herbal tea blends. Fruits not only contribute to the flavor but also infuse the tea with natural sweetness, reducing the need for added sweeteners. Citrus elements, in particular, can bring a refreshing zest to the blend.

Understanding Herbal Properties:

Each herb carries its unique set of properties, whether it's calming, energizing, or immune-boosting. Understanding the therapeutic benefits of herbs allows you to create blends tailored to specific needs. For example, combining chamomile and lavender for a calming bedtime blend or blending ginger and turmeric for an immune-boosting infusion.

Experimentation and Personalization:

The art of herbal tea blending is an ongoing journey of experimentation. Don't be afraid to mix and match different herbs to discover new and exciting combinations. Keep notes on the ratios and combinations that work well for your taste buds and wellness goals, allowing you to personalize your tea blends.

The art of blending herbal teas is a creative and rewarding endeavor. By mastering the basic principles of herbal tea blending—selecting base herbs, balancing flavors, incorporating aromatics, adding fruits, and understanding herbal properties—you can craft unique and flavorful blends that cater to your preferences and promote holistic well-being. So, grab your favorite herbs and embark on a journey of sensory discovery through the world of herbal tea blending.

Creating Balanced and
Flavorful Blends

The art of blending is a delicate dance of flavors, aromas, and textures, where a skilled craftsman transforms individual elements into a harmonious composition. Whether it's the world of perfumery, tea, coffee, spirits, or culinary delights, blending is a centuries-old practice that requires precision, intuition, and a keen understanding of the ingredients involved. In this exploration, we delve into the nuances of blending, uncovering the secrets behind creating balanced and flavorful blends that captivate the senses.

Understanding the Elements:

Ingredient Selection:

The foundation of a great blend lies in the careful selection of high-quality ingredients. Each component contributes its unique characteristics, and the blender must be attuned to the subtleties of flavors and aromas. Whether it's the robustness of coffee beans, the complexity of spices, or the nuances of essential oils, choosing the right ingredients is the first step towards a successful blend.

The Role of Base, Middle, and Top Notes:

Just like in perfumery, where scents are categorized into base, middle, and top notes, blending in various realms follows a similar principle. In tea, for instance, the base notes might come from a bold black tea, complemented by the milder middle notes of green tea, and topped off with the aromatic high notes of herbs or flowers. Understanding the role of each note is pivotal in achieving a well-rounded blend.

The Artistic Process:

Precision and Consistency:

Achieving a consistent blend requires precision in measurement and an unwavering commitment to quality. Whether it's measuring coffee beans to the gram or ensuring a consistent ratio of spices, the art of blending demands meticulous attention to detail.

Experimentation and Innovation:

Blenders are akin to artists, experimenting with different combinations to discover new and exciting flavors. Innovation plays a crucial role in the blending process, pushing boundaries and creating blends that surprise and delight the palate.

Creating Balance:
Balancing Flavor Profiles:

A successful blend is one where no single element overpowers the others. Achieving a balanced flavor profile involves a delicate interplay of sweetness, bitterness, acidity, and other taste components. The artful blender understands how to adjust these elements to create a seamless and enjoyable experience.

Texture and Mouthfeel:

Beyond taste, texture and mouthfeel contribute significantly to the overall sensory experience. Whether it's the velvety smoothness of a well-blended whiskey or the satisfying crunch in a spice mix, considering the tactile aspects enhances the art of blending.

The art of blending is a timeless craft that transcends various industries, each with its unique set of challenges and opportunities. From the symphony of flavors in a gourmet dish to the captivating aroma of a signature perfume, blending is the alchemy that transforms ordinary ingredients into extraordinary creations. To master the art of blending is to embark on a journey of sensory exploration, where creativity, expertise, and passion converge to produce blends that leave a lasting impression on those fortunate enough to experience them.

Exploring Aromas and Tastes for Maximum Wellness

In the intricate world of flavors and fragrances, the art of blending takes center stage, offering a sensory journey that goes beyond the ordinary. This ancient practice has evolved into a contemporary pursuit, transcending culinary boundaries to embrace a holistic approach to well-being. The art of blending not only tantalizes our taste buds but also engages our sense of smell, creating a symphony of aromas and tastes that contribute to maximum wellness.

Aromatherapy and Flavor Fusion:

At the heart of the art of blending lies the harmonious union of aromatherapy and flavor fusion. Aromatherapy, the therapeutic use of aromatic compounds, has been revered for its ability to influence mood and promote relaxation. When seamlessly integrated with culinary endeavors, it elevates the dining experience to new heights. By selecting and combining essential oils or natural extracts, one can create a myriad of aromatic profiles that stimulate the senses and enhance overall well-being.

In the realm of flavor fusion, blending is an art form that transcends traditional recipes. Experimenting with herbs, spices, and complementary ingredients allows for the creation of unique taste profiles. The careful balance of sweet, salty, sour, bitter, and umami flavors not only satisfies the palate but also contributes to a holistic and well-rounded eating experience.

Tea Blending: An Ancient Tradition Reimagined:

Tea, with its rich history spanning centuries and diverse cultures, has long been a canvas for the art of blending. Today, tea enthusiasts are rediscovering the joy of crafting personalized blends by combining various tea leaves, herbs, fruits, and spices. From calming chamomile and invigorating peppermint to antioxidant-rich green tea and zesty citrus, the possibilities are endless. Tea blending is more than a sensory delight; it's a mindful practice that encourages exploration and self-discovery.

Health Benefits of Blending:

Beyond the pleasure of savoring unique combinations, the art of blending contributes to our overall well-being. The intentional selection of ingredients allows for the incorporation of health-promoting elements into our diets. From anti-inflammatory spices to immune-boosting herbs, blending becomes a conscious choice to support physical health and vitality.

Mindful Blending for Personalized Wellness:
The art of blending extends beyond the kitchen and tea table; it encompasses a holistic approach to wellness. Mindful blending encourages individuals to tune into their own preferences, allowing for the creation of blends that resonate with personal tastes and health goals. Whether through herbal infusions, culinary creations, or aromatic experiences, the act of blending becomes a form of self-care, promoting balance and harmony in daily life.

In the pursuit of maximum wellness, the art of blending emerges as a sensory journey that engages the body, mind, and spirit. From the vibrant world of culinary concoctions to the soothing embrace of aromatic blends, the possibilities are as diverse as the ingredients themselves. As we delve into the art of blending, we not only discover new flavors and fragrances but also unlock a pathway to holistic well-being, one blend at a time.

CHAPTER 3: NOURISHING INFUSIONS FOR WELLNESS

Herbal Teas for Immune Support

In the quest for optimal health and well-being, many individuals are turning to natural remedies to fortify their immune systems. Herbal teas have long been celebrated for their therapeutic properties, offering a delightful and soothing way to support overall wellness. Let's explore a selection of herbal infusions known for their immune-boosting benefits and how they can play a crucial role in nourishing your body.

Echinacea Elixir:

Echinacea is renowned for its immune-stimulating properties. The roots and flowers of this purple coneflower are often brewed into a robust tea, creating a fragrant elixir that may help prevent and alleviate the symptoms of the common cold. Regular consumption of Echinacea tea can provide your immune system with the support it needs to ward off infections.

Ginger and Turmeric Tonic:

Ginger and turmeric are a dynamic duo known for their anti-inflammatory and antioxidant properties. Combining these two powerhouse roots in a soothing herbal tea can help reduce inflammation in the body, support digestion, and contribute to overall immune function. Add a hint of lemon and honey for a delightful flavor boost.

Chamomile and Lemon Balm Bliss:

Chamomile and lemon balm are renowned for their calming effects on the nervous system, promoting relaxation and reducing stress. Stress reduction is essential for a robust immune system. This gentle and aromatic tea not only supports your body in unwinding but also contributes to a strengthened immune response.

Nettle Leaf Nectar:

Nettle leaf tea is rich in vitamins and minerals, making it a nourishing infusion for overall health. Its immune-boosting properties are attributed to the presence of antioxidants and anti-inflammatory compounds. Nettle tea can be a wonderful addition to your wellness routine, providing essential nutrients that support your body's defense mechanisms.

Licorice Root Lullaby:

Licorice root is not only sweet in flavor but also packs a punch in immune-boosting potential. This tea has antiviral and anti-inflammatory properties, making it a valuable ally during times of seasonal challenges. Be mindful of the potential effects on blood pressure and consult with a healthcare professional if you have any concerns.

Holy Basil Harmony:

Also known as Tulsi, holy basil is revered in Ayurvedic medicine for its adaptogenic properties. Holy basil tea can help the body adapt to stress, while its antibacterial and antiviral qualities contribute to a strengthened immune system. Enjoy a cup of holy basil tea to foster a sense of balance and well-being.

Incorporating nourishing herbal infusions into your daily routine can be a delicious and effective way to support your immune system. Whether you're sipping on Echinacea elixir, enjoying a ginger and turmeric tonic, or indulging in a chamomile and lemon balm bliss, these herbal teas offer a holistic approach to wellness. As with any health regimen, it's essential to consult with a healthcare professional to ensure that these herbal infusions align with your individual health needs. Embrace the healing power of nature and make herbal teas a comforting and health-enhancing ritual in your life.

Infusions to Boost Energy and Vitality

In our fast-paced lives, maintaining optimal energy levels and vitality is crucial for overall well-being. While a balanced diet and regular exercise are fundamental, incorporating nourishing infusions into your daily routine can provide an extra boost of essential nutrients and promote wellness. Let's explore some invigorating infusions that can enhance your energy and vitality naturally.

Green Tea Elixir:

Green tea is renowned for its rich antioxidant content, particularly catechins and polyphenols. These compounds have been associated with improved metabolism and enhanced energy levels. Create a refreshing green tea elixir by steeping high-quality green tea leaves in hot water. Add a touch of honey and a slice of lemon for a burst of flavor and an additional vitamin C boost.

Ginger Zest Infusion:

Ginger is celebrated for its anti-inflammatory properties and ability to stimulate circulation. Prepare a ginger zest infusion by steeping fresh ginger slices in hot water. Ginger can help alleviate fatigue and boost energy levels, making it an excellent choice for those looking to add a spicy kick to their wellness routine.

Citrus Burst Herbal Blend:

Citrus fruits like oranges and lemons are rich in vitamin C, a powerful antioxidant that supports the immune system and combats fatigue. Create a citrus burst herbal infusion by combining citrus

slices with herbs like mint or basil. This infusion
not only revitalizes your senses but also provides
a hydrating and vitamin-packed elixir.

Turmeric and Honey Fusion:

Turmeric contains curcumin, known for its
anti-inflammatory and antioxidant properties.
Create a warming infusion by steeping turmeric
slices or powder in hot water. Add a dollop of
honey for sweetness and additional health
benefits. This infusion can help reduce
inflammation, promote digestion, and contribute
to overall vitality.

Hibiscus Berry Bliss:

Hibiscus flowers are not only visually appealing
but also packed with antioxidants and vitamin C.
Combine hibiscus petals with a mix of berries
like blueberries and strawberries for a flavorful

infusion. The result is a delightful hibiscus berry bliss that not only supports energy levels but also contributes to heart health.

Minty Fresh Revitalizer:
Mint is known for its invigorating aroma and digestive properties. Create a minty fresh infusion by steeping fresh mint leaves in hot water. This infusion can help soothe the digestive system, reduce stress, and promote mental clarity—qualities that are essential for overall well-being and vitality.

Incorporating nourishing infusions into your daily routine is a simple yet effective way to boost energy and vitality naturally. These infusions not only provide a delightful alternative to sugary beverages but also offer a range of health benefits. Experiment with different combinations and find the infusion that suits your taste buds while enhancing your overall wellness. Cheers to a revitalized and energized you!

Calming Blends for Stress Relief

In the fast-paced and often demanding world we live in, finding moments of tranquility and stress relief is essential for overall well-being. One effective and natural way to promote relaxation and nourish your body is through calming blends of infusions. These nourishing infusions not only provide a delightful sensory experience but also offer a range of health benefits that can contribute to your overall wellness. Let's explore some calming blends specifically crafted for stress relief:

1. Chamomile and Lavender Harmony:
Ingredients: Chamomile flowers, dried lavender buds.

Benefits: Chamomile is renowned for its calming properties, promoting relaxation and aiding in sleep. Lavender complements chamomile with its soothing aroma and potential anxiety-reducing effects.

2. Minty Serenity Elixir:

Ingredients: Peppermint leaves, spearmint leaves.

Benefits: Mint has a refreshing quality that can help alleviate tension and promote a sense of calm. It is also known for its digestive benefits, contributing to overall well-being.

3. Lemon Balm and Valerian Dreamtime Blend:

Ingredients: Lemon balm leaves, valerian root.

Benefits: Lemon balm is often used to reduce stress and anxiety, while valerian root is known for its potential to improve sleep quality. Together, they create a dreamy infusion perfect for winding down.

4. Rose and Passionflower Euphoria:

Ingredients: Dried rose petals, passionflower.

Benefits: Rose petals bring a touch of floral elegance while passionflower is believed to have calming effects, potentially reducing anxiety and promoting a relaxed state of mind.

5. Ginger Zen Fusion:

Ingredients: Fresh ginger slices, lemongrass.

Benefits: Ginger is known for its anti-inflammatory properties and can help soothe the digestive system. Lemongrass adds a citrusy note, contributing to a refreshing and uplifting infusion.

Brewing Tips:

Use fresh, high-quality ingredients for the best flavor and therapeutic benefits.

Steep the infusions in hot water for at least 5-7 minutes to extract the full range of flavors and health-promoting compounds.

Experiment with honey or a splash of lemon for added taste and immune-boosting benefits.

Incorporating these calming blends into your daily routine can provide a moment of mindfulness and contribute to a healthier, more balanced life. Whether you enjoy them in the morning to start your day on a peaceful note or in the evening to unwind, these nourishing infusions can be a delightful addition to your wellness journey. Take a break, sip on a cup of tranquility, and let the stress melt away.

Chapter 4: Customizing Herbal Teas for Your Health Goals

Addressing Common Ailments with Herbal Teas

Introduction:

Herbal teas have been cherished for centuries as natural remedies for various health concerns. Whether you're seeking relaxation, immune support, or relief from common ailments, customizing herbal teas can be a delightful and effective way to promote well-being. In this guide, we'll explore the art of blending herbal teas to address common ailments and help you achieve your health goals.

Understanding the Power of Herbs:

Herbs have long been recognized for their therapeutic properties. Each herb possesses unique compounds that contribute to its medicinal qualities. By understanding the benefits of different herbs, you can tailor your herbal tea blends to target specific health concerns.

Relaxation and Stress Relief:

For those seeking relaxation and stress relief, consider incorporating calming herbs into your tea blend. Chamomile, lavender, and lemon balm are renowned for their soothing properties. These herbs can help relax the nervous system, promote better sleep, and alleviate stress and anxiety.

Immune Support:

To boost your immune system and ward off common illnesses, create a tea blend rich in immune-boosting herbs. Echinacea, elderberry, and ginger are excellent choices. These herbs are known for their ability to strengthen the immune response, providing added defense against colds and flu.

Digestive Health:

Herbal teas can also be customized to support digestive health. Peppermint, fennel, and ginger are renowned for their digestive benefits. These herbs can ease indigestion, reduce bloating, and alleviate symptoms of irritable bowel syndrome (IBS).

Respiratory Wellness:

For respiratory issues such as congestion or a persistent cough, consider blending herbs with expectorant and anti-inflammatory properties. Eucalyptus, thyme, and licorice root can help clear airways, reduce mucus, and soothe respiratory discomfort.

Combating Insomnia:

If you struggle with insomnia or poor sleep quality, crafting a bedtime herbal tea blend can be beneficial. Valerian root, passionflower, and chamomile are popular choices known for their calming effects, promoting restful sleep.

Combining Herbs for Holistic Benefits:

Experiment with combining different herbs to create well-rounded teas that address multiple health goals simultaneously. For example, a blend of peppermint, chamomile, and lemon balm can provide relaxation, digestive support, and a boost to the immune system all in one cup. Customizing herbal teas for your health goals is a delightful and holistic approach to well-being. By harnessing the natural power of herbs, you can address common ailments and promote overall health. Whether you're sipping a cup of tea to unwind after a long day or crafting a blend to support specific health needs, the world of herbal teas offers a diverse array of flavors and benefits to explore.

Tailoring Blends to Individual Wellness Needs

Herbal teas have been cherished for centuries as natural remedies to promote health and well-being. With a myriad of herbs available, each boasting unique properties, customizing herbal teas can be a powerful and personalized approach to address individual health goals. Whether you're seeking relaxation, immune support, or digestive harmony, crafting your own herbal blends allows you to tailor your tea to meet your specific wellness needs.

Understanding Herbal Properties:

Before diving into the art of customization, it's essential to familiarize yourself with the properties of different herbs. Some herbs, like chamomile and lavender, are renowned for their calming effects, making them ideal choices for those looking to unwind and manage stress. Meanwhile, ginger and peppermint are known for their digestive benefits, aiding in digestion and alleviating discomfort. By understanding these properties, you can select herbs that align with your health objectives.

Personalized Blends for Wellness Goals: Stress Relief Blend:

Chamomile: Known for its calming properties, chamomile helps reduce stress and anxiety.

Lavender: Adds a soothing aroma and complements chamomile in promoting relaxation.

Immune Support Blend:

Echinacea: Renowned for its immune-boosting properties, echinacea can help fend off colds and infections.

Elderberry: Packed with antioxidants, elderberry supports the immune system and may reduce the duration of colds.

Digestive Harmony Blend:

Ginger: Eases nausea and supports digestion by reducing inflammation.

Peppermint: Known for its ability to soothe the digestive tract and alleviate indigestion.

Energy and Focus Blend:

Ginseng: Enhances mental clarity and provides a natural energy boost.

Rosemary: Known for its cognitive benefits, rosemary can improve focus and concentration.

Detox Blend:

Dandelion: Supports liver function and aids in detoxification.

Nettle: Acts as a diuretic, helping to flush out toxins from the body.

Brewing Techniques:

The art of herbal tea customization extends beyond ingredient selection to brewing techniques. Experiment with steeping times, water temperatures, and ratios to find the perfect balance for your desired effects. For example, longer steeping times generally extract more medicinal compounds, while shorter times result in a milder flavor.

Safety Considerations:

While herbal teas can offer numerous health benefits, it's crucial to be aware of potential interactions with medications and individual sensitivities. Consult with a healthcare professional if you have any concerns, especially if you are pregnant, nursing, or taking medications.

Customizing herbal teas for your health goals is a delightful and empowering journey. By combining the right herbs and understanding their properties, you can create blends that cater to your unique wellness needs. Whether you seek relaxation, immune support, digestive harmony, or increased energy, the world of herbal teas provides a diverse palette to support your health and well-being.

Combining Herbs for Maximum Health Benefits

Herbal teas have been valued for centuries for their therapeutic properties and ability to promote overall well-being. Customizing your herbal teas to align with your specific health goals allows you to harness the maximum benefits of various herbs. Whether you're aiming to boost immunity, improve digestion, or enhance relaxation, the right combination of herbs can make a significant difference. Let's explore the art of crafting personalized herbal teas tailored to your unique health needs.

Understanding Individual Herbs:

Before delving into combinations, it's crucial to understand the properties of individual herbs. Some herbs are known for their calming effects, such as chamomile and lavender, while others, like ginger and peppermint, are praised for their digestive benefits. Research and familiarize yourself with the specific properties of herbs to make informed choices when blending.

Immunity-Boosting Blends:

For those looking to strengthen their immune system, consider combining herbs with potent immune-boosting properties. Echinacea, elderberry, and astragalus are renowned for their ability to enhance the body's natural defenses. Mixing these herbs with a touch of antioxidant-rich green tea creates a powerful blend that supports overall immune health.

Digestive Harmony:

If digestive health is a priority, create a blend that includes soothing herbs like peppermint, ginger, and fennel. Peppermint aids in relieving indigestion, ginger supports digestion and reduces nausea, while fennel helps alleviate bloating. Combining these herbs provides a harmonious and effective solution for digestive discomfort.

Stress Relief and Relaxation:

To promote relaxation and reduce stress, turn to calming herbs such as chamomile, lavender, and lemon balm. Chamomile is renowned for its calming properties, lavender contributes to relaxation, and lemon balm helps alleviate anxiety. This combination creates a delightful and tranquil tea to unwind after a hectic day.

Energy-Boosting Elixirs:

Crafting a tea blend for an energy boost involves selecting invigorating herbs like ginseng, ginkgo biloba, and yerba mate. These herbs are known for their ability to enhance mental alertness and combat fatigue. Adding a hint of citrusy herbs like lemon verbena can provide a refreshing and revitalizing touch.

Anti-Inflammatory Infusions:

For those seeking anti-inflammatory benefits, consider combining turmeric, ginger, and cinnamon. Turmeric contains curcumin, a potent anti-inflammatory compound, while ginger and cinnamon contribute to overall well-being and add a delightful flavor profile. This blend not only supports inflammation reduction but also offers a warm and comforting experience.

Balancing Hormones Naturally:

Certain herbs, like red clover, licorice, and dong quai, are known for their potential to balance hormones naturally. Crafting a tea blend with these herbs may offer support for menstrual health and hormonal balance. Consult with a healthcare professional before incorporating such blends regularly.

Customizing herbal teas for your health goals allows you to create a personalized and enjoyable wellness routine. By understanding the properties of individual herbs and experimenting with various combinations, you can craft teas that cater to your specific needs. Whether you're aiming to boost immunity, improve digestion, or enhance relaxation, the world of herbal teas offers a myriad of possibilities for optimizing your health and well-being.

CHAPTER 5: RITUALS AND PRACTICES

Incorporating Herbal Teas into Daily Routines

In the fast-paced world we live in, finding moments of tranquility and self-care is essential for maintaining a healthy and balanced life. One way to incorporate mindfulness into daily routines is by embracing the ancient practice of herbal tea consumption. Beyond being a comforting beverage, herbal teas can become a ritualistic part of your day, offering a myriad of health benefits. In this article, we'll explore the art of incorporating herbal teas into daily routines and the positive impact it can have on overall well-being.

Morning Serenity:

Begin your day with a sense of calm by establishing a morning tea ritual. Replace your regular cup of coffee with a soothing herbal blend. Options like chamomile, peppermint, or ginger tea can awaken your senses without the jitters associated with caffeine. Take a few moments to savor the warmth, inhale the fragrant steam, and set positive intentions for the day ahead.

Midday Rejuvenation:

As the day unfolds, find a moment to pause and rejuvenate. Herbal teas like hibiscus or green tea can provide a refreshing pick-me-up while offering antioxidants and supporting hydration. Create a brief ritual around your tea break, perhaps by stepping outside for some fresh air, allowing your mind to reset and recharge.

Afternoon Focus:

Combat the afternoon slump with herbal teas that enhance mental clarity and focus. Herbs like rosemary, ginkgo biloba, or lemon balm can be brewed into a delightful infusion. Establish a tea-drinking routine during your work hours, creating a mindful space for concentration and productivity.

Evening Relaxation:

Wind down your day with a calming evening ritual. Opt for herbal teas known for their relaxing properties, such as lavender, chamomile, or valerian root. Enjoy your tea in a quiet space, away from screens, to signal to your body that it's time to unwind. This ritual can pave the way for a restful night's sleep.

Social Connection:

Herbal teas also make for a wonderful addition to social rituals. Invite friends or family to join you in a tea ceremony, fostering meaningful connections. Share the experience of trying new blends or creating personalized tea blends together, making it a memorable and shared ritual.

Custom Blends and Personalized Rituals:

Experiment with creating your own herbal tea blends, tailoring them to your specific needs. Whether it's a blend for relaxation, energy, or immune support, crafting your teas adds a personal touch to the ritual. Consider incorporating elements like dried flowers, herbs, or spices for a sensory experience.

Incorporating herbal teas into daily routines is more than just a beverage choice; it's a mindful practice that promotes overall wellness. By infusing your day with intentional moments centered around herbal teas, you cultivate a sense of balance, tranquility, and connection with yourself and the world around you. Embrace the ritual, savor the flavors, and let the simple act of enjoying herbal teas become a cornerstone of your well-being journey.

Mindful Tea Drinking for Enhanced Well-Being

In a world that often moves at a frenetic pace, finding moments of peace and mindfulness is essential for maintaining overall well-being. One such ancient practice that offers a perfect blend of tranquility and taste is mindful tea drinking. Rooted in various cultures across the globe, the art of sipping tea mindfully has been celebrated not only for its rich flavors but also for its potential to enhance mental clarity, reduce stress, and promote a sense of well-being.

The Ritual of Preparation:

Mindful tea drinking begins with the thoughtful preparation of the tea itself. Selecting high-quality tea leaves or herbs is crucial, as the fragrance and taste play a pivotal role in the experience. The ritualistic preparation process, whether it involves brewing loose leaves or preparing a traditional matcha ceremony, sets the stage for a mindful journey.

Choosing the Right Tea:

Opt for high-quality, organic tea leaves or herbs to ensure a pure and authentic experience.

Experiment with various types, such as green, black, white, or herbal teas, to find the flavors that resonate with you.

Mindful Brewing:

Pay attention to the water temperature and steeping time for each type of tea to unlock its full potential.

Engage your senses by inhaling the aroma of the tea as it brews, fostering a connection with the present moment.

The Art of Serving:

Mindful tea drinking involves more than just sipping; it encompasses the entire process, from pouring to savoring.

Delicate Pouring:

Pour the tea with intention, allowing the warm liquid to fill the cup gracefully.

Observe the color of the tea, appreciating its nuances and subtleties.

Engaging the Senses:

Feel the warmth of the cup in your hands, fostering a tactile connection.

Take a moment to admire the appearance of the tea, observing the way it dances and shimmers in the light.

The Mindful Sip:

The actual act of sipping the tea becomes a meditation in itself, requiring full attention to the present moment.

Savoring Each Sip:

Take small, deliberate sips, allowing the flavors to unfold on your palate.
Notice the temperature and texture of the tea as it lingers in your mouth.

Mindful Breathing:

Sync your breath with each sip, creating a rhythmic and calming experience.
Allow any intrusive thoughts to pass, focusing on the sensory experience of the tea.

Benefits of Mindful Tea Drinking:

Stress Reduction:

The act of mindful tea drinking promotes relaxation, helping to alleviate stress and anxiety.

Increased Awareness:

By engaging the senses and focusing on the present moment, tea drinking enhances overall awareness and mindfulness.

Cultural Connection:

Exploring various tea traditions connects individuals to rich cultural practices, fostering a sense of unity and understanding.

In a world that often rushes by, the practice of mindful tea drinking offers a sanctuary of serenity. Through the careful selection, preparation, and savoring of tea, individuals can elevate a simple daily activity into a transformative ritual, promoting enhanced well-being and a deeper connection to the present moment. Embrace the art of mindful tea drinking and allow it to become a cherished part of your daily routine, enriching both your palate and your soul.

Sharing the Healing Power of Herbal Teas with Others

In the fast-paced world we inhabit, finding moments of tranquility and connection has become essential for our well-being. One ancient practice that continues to offer solace and healing is the age-old tradition of brewing and sharing herbal teas. Rooted in diverse cultures and cherished for their therapeutic properties, herbal teas provide not only physical benefits but also foster a sense of community and shared well-being.

The Healing Power of Herbal Teas:

Herbal teas, concocted from a variety of leaves, flowers, roots, and spices, have been used for centuries to address various health concerns. Whether it's the calming effects of chamomile, the immune-boosting properties of echinacea, or the digestion-soothing benefits of peppermint, each herbal infusion carries a unique blend of nutrients and compounds that contribute to overall health.

The Ritualistic Experience:

Brewing and enjoying herbal teas is a ritual that goes beyond the mere act of consumption. The process of selecting herbs, measuring ingredients, and patiently waiting for the infusion creates a space for mindfulness and introspection. The aromatic steam rising from the cup becomes a sensory experience, calming the mind and preparing it for the moment of sipping and savoring.

Sharing the Experience:

The beauty of herbal tea rituals lies in their ability to be shared. Bringing people together over a pot of carefully brewed herbal tea fosters a sense of community and connection. Whether it's a cozy family gathering, an intimate conversation with friends, or a communal wellness event, the act of sharing herbal teas becomes a vehicle for the exchange of warmth, comfort, and healing energy.

Creating a Herbal Tea Community:

To amplify the benefits of herbal teas, individuals are increasingly coming together to form herbal tea communities. These communities serve as spaces for enthusiasts to share their knowledge, experiences, and favorite blends. Through workshops, tastings, and collaborative events, participants not only expand their understanding of herbal teas but also forge meaningful connections with like-minded individuals.

Promoting Wellness and Mindfulness:

Beyond the physical health benefits, herbal tea rituals encourage mindfulness and self-care. Taking a pause in our hectic lives to engage in a deliberate, soothing practice helps cultivate a deeper connection with oneself and the world. The aromatic symphony of herbs and spices becomes a meditative experience, promoting mental clarity and emotional well-being.

In a world that often seems to move at an overwhelming pace, rituals and practices centered around herbal teas offer a sanctuary for healing and connection. Embracing the art of brewing and sharing herbal teas not only enhances our physical well-being but also nurtures our collective need for community, mindfulness, and moments of tranquility. As we continue to explore and celebrate the diverse world of herbal teas, we find ourselves on a journey towards a more balanced and harmonious existence.

CONCLUSION

Healing Herbal Tea Bible: Preparing Nourishing is a comprehensive and insightful guide that transcends the boundaries of a typical herbal tea book. Authored with precision and passion, this literary masterpiece not only delves into the rich history of herbal infusions but also empowers readers with the knowledge and skills necessary to harness the healing potential of herbs for enhanced well-being.

One of the remarkable aspects of this book is its meticulous approach to blending traditional wisdom with contemporary science. The author skillfully navigates the vast landscape of herbal teas, providing readers with a treasure trove of information on the medicinal properties of various herbs. The emphasis on mastering the art of preparation is particularly commendable, as it elevates the book from a mere compendium of recipes to a guide that encourages a deeper connection with the healing power of nature.

The narrative unfolds seamlessly, guiding readers through the enchanting world of herbs and their therapeutic benefits. Each chapter is a testament to the author's dedication to fostering a holistic understanding of herbal teas, covering everything from the selection and cultivation of herbs to the artful blending of flavors for both pleasure and wellness. The book is not just a manual; it is a journey that invites readers to explore, experiment, and embrace the transformative potential of herbal teas.

Furthermore, the inclusion of practical tips and expert advice enhances the book's utility, making it accessible to both novice tea enthusiasts and seasoned herbalists. The author's expertise shines through, providing a reliable resource that encourages readers to embark on their own herbal tea journey with confidence. The detailed instructions on brewing techniques, the art of combining herbs, and the thoughtful consideration of individual preferences make this book an indispensable companion for anyone seeking to integrate herbal teas into their daily routine.

Beyond its instructional value, the "Healing Herbal Tea Bible" also succeeds in sparking an appreciation for the symbiotic relationship between nature and human well-being. The eloquent prose and vivid descriptions transport readers to herb gardens and tea ceremonies, fostering a sense of connection to the ancient traditions that have paved the way for our contemporary understanding of herbal medicine.

In a world where wellness is increasingly sought through natural means, this book emerges as a beacon of knowledge, guiding readers toward a path of self-discovery and vitality. It is not just a book about tea; it is a testament to the transformative potential that lies within the leaves, flowers, and roots of the plants that have been our companions throughout history.

In essence, "Healing Herbal Tea Bible" is a celebration of the therapeutic art of tea-making, an ode to the healing power of nature, and a timeless guide that will continue to inspire and enrich the lives of readers for generations to come. As the final page is turned, one is left with a profound sense of gratitude for the author's dedication to preserving and sharing the age-old wisdom encapsulated in the art of preparing nourishing herbal infusions. This book is not merely a read; it is an invitation to embark on a journey of wellness, vitality, and the enduring magic of herbal teas.